GASTRIC-HEALTH GUIDE

UNDERSTANDING AND OVERCOMING DIGESTIVE DISORDERS

THERESA P. JAMES MD.

TABLE OF CONTENT

Introduction

Overview of gastrointestinal disorders

Gastrointestinal disorders encompass a wide range of conditions that affect the digestive system, including the esophagus, stomach, intestines, liver, gallbladder, and pancreas. These disorders can vary in severity and may cause a variety of symptoms, ranging from mild discomfort to severe pain and disruption of daily life. Some of the most common gastrointestinal disorders include:

Gastro-Esophageal Reflux Disease (GERD):

GERD is a chronic condition characterized by the reflux of stomach acid into the esophagus, leading to symptoms such as heartburn, regurgitation, and difficulty swallowing.

Irritable Bowel Syndrome (IBS):

IBS is a functional gastrointestinal disorder characterized by abdominal pain, bloating, diarrhea, and/or constipation. Symptoms may vary in severity and often occur in response to triggers such as stress, certain foods, or hormonal changes.

Gastritis:

Gastritis refers to inflammation of the stomach lining, which can be acute or chronic. Common symptoms include abdominal pain, nausea, vomiting, bloating, and loss of appetite.

Celiac Disease:

Celiac disease is an autoimmune disorder triggered by the consumption of gluten, a protein found in wheat, barley, and rye. It causes damage to the small intestine, leading to malabsorption of nutrients and symptoms such as diarrhea, abdominal pain, bloating, and fatigue.

Crohn's Disease:

- Crohn's disease is a chronic inflammatory bowel disease that can affect any part of the digestive tract, from the mouth to the anus. Symptoms may include abdominal pain, diarrhea, weight loss, fatigue, and malnutrition.

Diverticulitis:

Diverticulitis occurs when small pouches (diverticula) in the colon become inflamed or infected. Symptoms may include abdominal pain (usually in the lower left side), fever, nausea, vomiting, and changes in bowel habits.

Pancreatitis:

Pancreatitis is inflammation of the pancreas, which can be acute or chronic. It causes severe abdominal pain, nausea, vomiting, and fever. Chronic pancreatitis can lead to long-term complications such as diabetes and pancreatic insufficiency.

These are just a few examples of gastrointestinal disorders, and there are many other conditions that can affect the digestive system. Treatment for these disorders often involves a combination of lifestyle modifications, medications, dietary changes, and, in some cases, surgery. Management of gastrointestinal disorders typically requires a multidisciplinary approach involving healthcare providers such as gastroenterologists, dietitians, and mental health professionals. Early diagnosis and proper management are essential for improving symptoms and quality of life for individuals living with these conditions.

Importance of understanding and managing these conditions

Understanding and managing gastrointestinal conditions are crucial for several reasons:

1. Improved Quality of Life: Effective management strategies can help alleviate symptoms and improve overall well-being, allowing individuals to lead more comfortable and fulfilling lives.

2. Prevention of Complications: Left untreated or poorly managed, gastrointestinal disorders can lead to complications such as esophageal ulcers, intestinal strictures, malnutrition, or even colon cancer. Understanding these conditions and implementing appropriate management strategies can help prevent or minimize the risk of complications.

3. Reduction of Symptoms: By understanding triggers and adopting lifestyle modifications, individuals can often reduce the frequency and severity of symptoms associated with gastrointestinal disorders, such as abdominal pain, bloating, diarrhea, or constipation.

4. Maintenance of Nutritional Health: Many gastrointestinal disorders can impact nutrient absorption or lead to dietary restrictions.

Managing these conditions effectively involves ensuring adequate nutrition to prevent deficiencies and maintain overall health.

5. Preservation of Mental Health: Living with chronic gastrointestinal conditions can take a toll on mental health, leading to stress, anxiety, and depression. Understanding the condition and having effective management strategies in place can help individuals cope better with the emotional challenges associated with their illness.

6. Optimal Treatment Outcomes: A thorough understanding of gastrointestinal disorders allows healthcare providers to tailor treatment plans to the individual needs of patients, leading to better treatment outcomes and potentially reducing the need for invasive procedures or hospitalizations.

7. Empowerment and Self-Advocacy: When individuals understand their condition and how it affects their body, they are better equipped to advocate for themselves in healthcare settings, ask informed questions, and actively participate in decision-making regarding their treatment and care.

Overall, understanding and managing gastrointestinal conditions are essential for improving quality of life, preventing complications, reducing symptoms, maintaining nutritional health, preserving mental well-being, achieving optimal treatment outcomes, and empowering individuals to take control of their health.

Purpose of the book: To provide information and practical tips for managing symptoms and improving quality of life

The purpose of this book is to serve as a comprehensive guide for individuals grappling with gastrointestinal disorders, offering not just information but also practical strategies to effectively manage symptoms and enhance their overall quality of life. In recognizing the often daunting and multifaceted nature of these conditions, the book aims to provide a beacon of knowledge and support for readers navigating the complexities of their digestive health.

Central to the book's mission is the provision of accurate and accessible information about various gastrointestinal disorders, ensuring readers gain a thorough understanding of their specific condition and its impact on their body.

By demystifying medical jargon and breaking down complex concepts into digestible pieces, the book empowers individuals to become informed advocates for their own health, enabling them to better comprehend the intricacies of their diagnosis, treatment options, and potential outcomes.

Moreover, the book goes beyond mere education by offering practical tips and strategies tailored to the unique needs and challenges posed by gastrointestinal disorders. From dietary modifications and lifestyle adjustments to stress management techniques and coping strategies, readers are equipped with a toolkit of evidence-based approaches aimed at alleviating symptoms and fostering holistic well-being. By emphasizing proactive self-care and empowerment, the book encourages readers to take an active role in managing their condition and optimizing their health outcomes.

Crucially, the book acknowledges the profound impact that gastrointestinal disorders can have on individuals' lives, extending beyond physical symptoms to encompass emotional, social, and psychological dimensions. Through compassionate and empathetic guidance, readers are supported in navigating the emotional complexities and practical obstacles that accompany chronic illness, fostering resilience, self-compassion, and a sense of community among those facing similar challenges.

Ultimately, this book serves as a beacon of hope and empowerment for individuals grappling with gastrointestinal disorders, offering not just information and practical tips but also a source of validation, support, and encouragement on their journey toward improved health and well-being. By fostering a sense of agency, resilience, and community, the book seeks to inspire readers to embrace their own capacity for healing and embark on a path toward a brighter, more vibrant future.

CHAPTER ONE: Understanding Gastrointestinal Disorders

GERD

Gastro-Esophageal Reflux Disease (GERD) is a chronic digestive disorder characterized by the reflux of stomach acid into the esophagus. This occurs due to a weakened or dysfunctional lower esophageal sphincter (LES), the muscular valve that separates the esophagus from the stomach.

Common symptoms of Gastro-Esophageal Reflux disease (GERD) include;

1. Heartburn: A burning sensation in the chest, often after eating or when lying down.
2. Regurgitation: Sour or bitter-tasting fluid that backs up into the throat or mouth.
3. Chest pain: Discomfort or pressure in the chest, sometimes mistaken for a heart attack.
4. Difficulty swallowing: Sensation of food getting stuck in the throat or chest.

5. Acidic taste in the mouth: Sour taste due to stomach acid backing up into the esophagus.
6. Sore throat: Irritation or inflammation of the throat caused by acid reflux.
7. Chronic cough: Persistent cough, especially at night, due to irritation of the throat or lungs.

Common triggers for GERD symptoms include:

1. Certain foods and beverages: Spicy foods, acidic foods (e.g., citrus fruits, tomatoes), fatty foods, caffeine, alcohol, and carbonated beverages can trigger or exacerbate symptoms.
2. Large meals: Overeating or consuming large meals can increase pressure on the stomach and contribute to reflux.
3. Eating before bedtime: Lying down shortly after eating can allow stomach acid to flow back into the esophagus more easily.
4. Tight clothing: Tight belts or waistbands can put pressure on the abdomen and contribute to reflux symptoms.
5. Smoking: Tobacco use can relax the lower esophageal sphincter (LES), allowing stomach acid to reflux into the esophagus.
6. Obesity: Excess weight, especially around the abdomen, can increase pressure on the stomach and LES, leading to reflux.

7. Medications: Certain medications, such as nonsteroidal anti-inflammatory drugs (NSAIDs), calcium channel blockers, and bisphosphonates, may relax the LES or irritate the esophagus, contributing to reflux symptoms.
Identifying and avoiding triggers can help manage GERD symptoms effectively.

Diagnostic Process and Treatment available

Diagnosis of Gastro-Esophageal Reflux disease (GERD) typically involves a combination of medical history, symptom evaluation, and diagnostic tests. Treatment options aim to alleviate symptoms, heal esophageal damage, and prevent complications. Here's an overview:

Diagnosis:

1. Medical History and Symptom Evaluation: Your healthcare provider will inquire about your symptoms, including heartburn, regurgitation, chest pain, difficulty swallowing, and other related issues. They may also ask about your diet, lifestyle habits, and medication use.

2. Physical Examination: A physical examination may be performed to assess for signs of GERD, such as abdominal tenderness or a hiatal hernia.

3. Diagnostic Tests:
   - Upper Endoscopy: A flexible tube with a camera (endoscope) is inserted through the mouth to examine the esophagus, stomach, and upper part of the small intestine. This allows for visualization of esophageal inflammation, ulcers, or other abnormalities.
   - Esophageal pH Monitoring: Measures acid levels in the esophagus over a period of time to assess acid reflux episodes and their correlation with symptoms.
   - Esophageal Manometry: Measures the pressure and muscle contractions in the esophagus to evaluate esophageal function and assess for abnormalities.

Treatment:

1. Lifestyle Modifications:
   - Dietary Changes: Avoiding trigger foods and beverages such as fatty or spicy foods, caffeine, alcohol, and acidic foods can help reduce reflux symptoms.
   - Weight Management: Losing excess weight, if applicable, can decrease pressure on the abdomen and reduce reflux.

- Elevating the Head of the Bed: Sleeping with the head of the bed elevated can help prevent acid reflux during sleep.

2. Medications:
   - Antacids: Over-the-counter antacids (e.g., Tums, Rolaids) can neutralize stomach acid and provide temporary relief from heartburn.
   - H2 Blockers: Histamine-2 (H2) receptor antagonists (e.g., ranitidine, famotidine) reduce stomach acid production and can alleviate symptoms.
   - Proton Pump Inhibitors (PPIs): Prescription-strength medications (e.g., omeprazole, esomeprazole) inhibit stomach acid production more effectively than H2 blockers and are often used for more severe or persistent symptoms.

3. Surgical Interventions: In some cases, surgical procedures such as fundoplication may be recommended for patients with severe GERD who do not respond to other treatments.

4. Monitoring and Follow-up: Regular monitoring and follow-up with a healthcare provider are important to assess treatment effectiveness, manage symptoms, and monitor for potential complications.

It's important to work closely with a healthcare provider to develop a personalized treatment plan tailored to your individual needs and preferences. Lifestyle modifications and medications can often effectively manage symptoms and improve quality of life for individuals with GERD. However, if symptoms persist or worsen despite treatment, further evaluation and adjustments to the treatment plan may be necessary.

Irritable Bowel Syndrome

Irritable Bowel Syndrome (IBS) is a common functional gastrointestinal disorder characterized by a combination of symptoms including abdominal pain or discomfort, bloating, and changes in bowel habits such as diarrhea, constipation, or alternating between the two. The exact cause of IBS is not fully understood, but factors such as abnormal gut motility, visceral hypersensitivity, altered gut-brain axis communication, and psychological factors like stress may play a role. Symptoms of IBS can vary widely in frequency and severity, often triggered by certain foods, stress, hormonal changes, or other factors. Diagnosis is typically based on the presence of characteristic symptoms and the exclusion of other gastrointestinal conditions through medical evaluation. Treatment for IBS often involves a combination of dietary modifications (e.g., low FODMAP diet), stress management techniques, medications to alleviate specific symptoms (e.g., antispasmodics for abdominal pain, laxatives for constipation), and lifestyle changes aimed at improving overall gut health and quality of life.

Gastritis

Gastritis is a condition characterized by inflammation of the stomach lining, which can occur suddenly (acute gastritis) or develop over time (chronic gastritis). It can result from various factors such as infection with Helicobacter pylori bacteria, excessive alcohol consumption, long-term use of nonsteroidal anti-inflammatory drugs (NSAIDs), autoimmune disorders, or stress. Symptoms of gastritis may include abdominal pain or discomfort, nausea, vomiting, bloating, loss of appetite, and a feeling of fullness after eating. In some cases, gastritis may be asymptomatic. Diagnosis is typically made through a combination of medical history, physical examination, and diagnostic tests such as endoscopy, blood tests, or stool tests. Treatment aims to alleviate symptoms, reduce inflammation, and address the underlying cause. This may involve medications to reduce stomach acid production (e.g., proton pump inhibitors), antibiotics to eradicate H. pylori infection if present, avoiding irritants such as alcohol and NSAIDs, dietary modifications (e.g., avoiding spicy or acidic foods), and stress management techniques. Chronic gastritis may require long-term management to prevent complications such as stomach ulcers or an increased risk of stomach cancer.

Celiac Disease

Celiac disease is an autoimmune disorder triggered by the ingestion of gluten, a protein found in wheat, barley, and rye. In individuals with celiac disease, consumption of gluten leads to an immune reaction that damages the lining of the small intestine, specifically the villi, which are finger-like projections that aid in nutrient absorption. This damage can result in various gastrointestinal symptoms such as diarrhea, abdominal pain, bloating, and weight loss, as well as non-gastrointestinal symptoms such as fatigue, joint pain, skin rashes, and nutritional deficiencies.

Triggers: Gluten-containing foods (e.g., wheat, barley, rye), cross-contamination with gluten, certain medications, and stress.

Diagnosis of celiac disease typically involves blood tests to detect specific antibodies associated with the condition, followed by confirmation through an intestinal biopsy to assess the degree of damage to the small intestine. Treatment for celiac disease involves strict adherence to a gluten-free diet, which involves avoiding all sources of gluten in food, beverages, medications, and personal care products. With proper dietary management, the intestinal lining can heal, and symptoms can improve over time.

It's important for individuals with celiac disease to work closely with healthcare providers, such as gastroenterologists and dietitians, to ensure proper diagnosis, ongoing management, and monitoring for potential complications such as nutritional deficiencies, osteoporosis, or other autoimmune disorders. Additionally, individuals with celiac disease should be vigilant about cross-contamination and regularly monitor their gluten-free diet to maintain optimal health and quality of life.

Crohn's disease

Crohn's disease is a chronic inflammatory bowel disease (IBD) characterized by inflammation of the digestive tract. It can affect any part of the gastrointestinal tract, from the mouth to the anus, but most commonly involves the small intestine and the beginning of the large intestine (colon). The exact cause of Crohn's disease is not fully understood, but it is thought to involve a combination of genetic, environmental, and immune system factors.

Symptoms

Symptoms of Crohn's disease can vary widely from person to person and may include abdominal pain, diarrhea, rectal bleeding, weight loss, fatigue, fever, and reduced appetite. In addition to gastrointestinal symptoms, Crohn's disease can also cause complications such as intestinal strictures (narrowing), fistulas (abnormal connections between organs), abscesses, and malnutrition due to poor nutrient absorption.

Triggers:

Specific foods (e.g., high-fat or high-fiber foods, spicy foods, dairy), stress, smoking, certain medications (e.g., nonsteroidal anti-inflammatory drugs), infections, and changes in the gut microbiome.

Diagnosis

Diagnosis of Crohn's disease typically involves a combination of medical history, physical examination, blood tests, imaging studies (such as CT scans or MRI), and endoscopic procedures (such as colonoscopy or upper endoscopy) to visualize the digestive tract and assess the extent of inflammation.

Treatment

Treatment for Crohn's disease aims to reduce inflammation, alleviate symptoms, and maintain remission. This often involves a combination of medications such as anti-inflammatory drugs (e.g., corticosteroids, mesalamine), immunomodulators (e.g., azathioprine, methotrexate), biologic therapies (e.g., anti-TNF agents), and symptom-specific medications (e.g., anti-diarrheal drugs). In some cases, surgery may be necessary to remove diseased portions of the intestine or address complications such as strictures or fistulas.

Additionally, lifestyle modifications such as dietary changes, stress management techniques, smoking cessation (as smoking can exacerbate Crohn's disease), and regular exercise may also be beneficial in managing symptoms and improving overall quality of life for individuals with Crohn's disease. Ongoing monitoring and management by a healthcare team, including gastroenterologists, dietitians, and other specialists, are essential for optimizing treatment outcomes and minimizing the risk of complications

Diverticulitis

Diverticulitis is a condition characterized by inflammation or infection of small pouches called diverticula that form in the lining of the colon, typically in the sigmoid colon, which is the lower part of the large intestine. Diverticula themselves are common and usually harmless, but when they become inflamed or infected, it can lead to symptoms and complications.

The exact cause of diverticulitis is not fully understood, but it is thought to involve a combination of factors, including increased pressure in the colon due to constipation or straining during bowel movements, as well as dietary factors such as a low-fiber diet.

Common symptoms of diverticulitis include:

1. Abdominal pain: Typically localized in the lower left side of the abdomen, although it can

occur on the right side or throughout the abdomen. The pain may be constant or intermittent and can range from mild to severe.

2. Fever: Often accompanies diverticulitis due to inflammation or infection.

3. Nausea and vomiting: Some individuals with diverticulitis may experience nausea or vomiting, especially if the condition is severe.

4. Changes in bowel habits: Diverticulitis can cause changes in bowel movements, such as diarrhea, constipation, or alternating between the two.

5. Abdominal tenderness: The abdomen may be tender to the touch, especially in the area where the diverticula are inflamed.

6. Bloating or gas: Some individuals with diverticulitis may experience bloating or increased gas production.

Common triggers for diverticulitis include:

1. Low-fiber diet: A diet low in fiber can lead to constipation and increased pressure in the colon, which may contribute to the formation of diverticula and increase the risk of diverticulitis.

2. Lack of physical activity: Sedentary lifestyle and lack of exercise can slow down bowel movements and increase the risk of

constipation, which may worsen diverticulitis symptoms.
3. Obesity: Excess weight, particularly around the abdomen, can increase pressure in the colon and contribute to the development or exacerbation of diverticulitis.
4. Aging: The risk of diverticulitis increases with age, with most cases occurring in individuals over 40 years old.
5. Genetics: Family history of diverticulitis or other gastrointestinal conditions may increase the risk of developing the condition.
6. Smoking: Tobacco use has been linked to an increased risk of diverticulitis.
7. Certain medications: Some medications, such as nonsteroidal anti-inflammatory drugs (NSAIDs) or steroids, may increase the risk of diverticulitis or exacerbate symptoms.

Diagnosis

Diagnosis of diverticulitis typically involves a combination of medical history, physical examination, blood tests (such as a complete blood count to check for signs of infection), and imaging studies (such as CT scans or ultrasound) to visualize the colon and confirm the presence of inflamed or infected diverticula.

Treatment:

Treatment for diverticulitis depends on the severity of symptoms and may include dietary modifications, antibiotics to treat infection, pain management, and in some cases, hospitalization for intravenous fluids and observation. In severe cases or for complications such as abscess formation, perforation, or bowel obstruction, surgery may be necessary to remove the affected portion of the colon.

Managing diverticulitis often involves dietary modifications, such as increasing fiber intake, staying hydrated, and avoiding foods that may trigger symptoms. In severe cases, treatment may include antibiotics, pain medication, and a clear liquid diet to rest the digestive system.

Prevention of diverticulitis and its complications often involves lifestyle modifications such as adopting a high-fiber diet to promote regular bowel movements and prevent constipation, staying hydrated, exercising regularly, and avoiding straining during bowel movements. Additionally, avoiding certain foods that may exacerbate symptoms, such as nuts, seeds, and popcorn, may be recommended for some individuals.

Regular monitoring and follow-up with a healthcare provider, particularly for individuals with a history of diverticulitis, can help prevent recurrence and manage the condition effectively.

Pancreatitis

Pancreatitis is inflammation of the pancreas, a gland located behind the stomach that plays a crucial role in digestion and blood sugar regulation. There are two main types of pancreatitis: acute pancreatitis, which occurs suddenly and usually resolves with treatment, and chronic pancreatitis, which is characterized by persistent inflammation and irreversible damage to the pancreas over time.

Acute pancreatitis is often triggered by factors such as gallstones, heavy alcohol consumption, certain medications, infections, trauma, or high levels of triglycerides in the blood. Symptoms of acute pancreatitis may include severe abdominal pain (often radiating to the back), nausea, vomiting, fever, rapid pulse, and tenderness in the abdomen. In severe cases, acute pancreatitis can lead to complications such as pancreatic necrosis (tissue death), pseudocysts (fluid-filled sacs), or organ failure.

Chronic pancreatitis, on the other hand, develops gradually and is often caused by long-term alcohol abuse, although other factors such as genetics, certain medical conditions, or recurrent episodes of acute pancreatitis may also contribute. Symptoms of chronic pancreatitis may include persistent abdominal pain, weight loss, oily or greasy stools (steatorrhea), diabetes mellitus due to impaired insulin production, and malnutrition due to poor digestion and nutrient absorption.

Common symptoms of pancreatitis include:

1. Abdominal pain: Typically located in the upper abdomen and may radiate to the back or chest. The pain can be severe and persistent, often described as dull, sharp, or burning.
2. Nausea and vomiting: Individuals with pancreatitis may experience nausea and vomiting, especially after eating or drinking.
3. Fever and chills: Fever may accompany pancreatitis, particularly if the inflammation is due to infection.

4. Rapid pulse: Increased heart rate may occur in response to pain or inflammation associated with pancreatitis.
5. Tender abdomen: The abdomen may be tender to the touch, particularly in the upper abdomen.
6. Jaundice: Yellowing of the skin and eyes may occur if pancreatitis affects the bile ducts and leads to obstruction of bile flow.
7. Changes in bowel habits: Pancreatitis can cause diarrhea or oily, foul-smelling stools (steatorrhea) due to impaired digestion and nutrient absorption.

Common triggers for pancreatitis include:

1. Gallstones: Obstruction of the pancreatic duct by gallstones is a common cause of acute pancreatitis.
2. Alcohol consumption: Heavy or chronic alcohol consumption is a leading cause of pancreatitis, particularly chronic pancreatitis.
3. High-fat diet: Consuming high-fat foods can stimulate the release of pancreatic enzymes, increasing the risk of pancreatitis, especially in individuals with gallstones or a history of pancreatitis.
4. Trauma or injury: Physical trauma to the abdomen, such as a car accident or severe blow, can lead to pancreatitis.

5. Certain medications: Some medications, such as corticosteroids, certain antibiotics, and immunosuppressants, may increase the risk of pancreatitis.
6. Infections: Viral infections such as mumps or bacterial infections in the pancreas can cause pancreatitis.
7. Genetic factors: Inherited conditions such as hereditary pancreatitis or cystic fibrosis can predispose individuals to pancreatitis.

Avoiding known triggers, such as excessive alcohol consumption and high-fat foods, maintaining a healthy lifestyle, managing underlying conditions, and seeking prompt medical attention for symptoms, can help reduce the risk of pancreatitis and its complications. Individuals with pancreatitis should work closely with healthcare providers to develop personalized treatment plans and lifestyle modifications to manage the condition effectively.

Diagnosis

Diagnosis of pancreatitis typically involves a combination of medical history, physical examination, blood tests (such as amylase and lipase levels to assess pancreatic enzyme levels), imaging studies (such as CT scans or MRI) to visualize the pancreas and assess for inflammation or other abnormalities, and sometimes endoscopic procedures (such as endoscopic ultrasound or ERCP) to evaluate the pancreas and surrounding structures more closely.

Treatment

Treatment for pancreatitis depends on the underlying cause and severity of symptoms. In cases of acute pancreatitis, treatment may involve hospitalization for pain management, intravenous fluids to prevent dehydration, nutritional support (often through a feeding tube), and monitoring for complications. Chronic pancreatitis may require ongoing management with pain medications, enzyme supplements to aid digestion, dietary modifications (such as a low-fat diet), and lifestyle changes (such as abstaining from alcohol).

In severe or recurrent cases of pancreatitis, surgery may be necessary to remove blockages in the pancreatic ducts, drain fluid collections or pseudocysts, or in some cases, remove part of the pancreas. Prevention of pancreatitis often involves avoiding known risk factors such as excessive alcohol consumption, maintaining a healthy weight, and managing conditions such as gallstones or high triglyceride levels effectively. Regular monitoring and follow-up with a healthcare provider are essential for individuals with pancreatitis to manage symptoms, prevent complications, and optimize their overall health and well-being.

Chapter TWO: Lifestyle Modifications for Better Digestive Health

Lifestyle modifications play a crucial role in promoting better digestive health, particularly in managing gastrointestinal disorders.

Importance of diet and nutrition in managing such conditions

Here's the importance of diet and nutrition in managing such conditions:

1. Reducing Trigger Foods: Certain foods and beverages can exacerbate symptoms of gastrointestinal disorders such as GERD, IBS, gastritis, celiac disease, and Crohn's disease. By identifying and avoiding trigger foods—such as spicy foods, acidic foods, caffeine, alcohol, high-fat foods, gluten-containing foods, and artificial sweeteners—individuals can minimize symptoms and improve their overall digestive health.

2. Increasing Fiber Intake: Adequate fiber intake is essential for maintaining regular bowel movements, preventing constipation, and promoting digestive health. For conditions

like diverticulitis and IBS, a high-fiber diet can help alleviate symptoms such as abdominal pain, bloating, and irregular bowel habits. However, individuals with certain gastrointestinal disorders, such as Crohn's disease or celiac disease, may need to tailor their fiber intake based on their specific needs and tolerances.

3. Balancing Macronutrients: Consuming a well-balanced diet that includes a variety of macronutrients—such as carbohydrates, proteins, and fats—is important for overall health and digestion. For example, individuals with pancreatitis may benefit from a low-fat diet to reduce strain on the pancreas, while those with celiac disease need to avoid gluten-containing grains like wheat, barley, and rye.

4. Hydration: Staying hydrated is essential for maintaining healthy digestion and preventing complications such as constipation. Drinking an adequate amount of water throughout the day helps keep stools soft and facilitates bowel movements. However, individuals with certain gastrointestinal disorders, such as GERD or gastroparesis, may need to adjust their fluid intake to avoid exacerbating symptoms.

5. Portion Control and Meal Timing: Eating smaller, more frequent meals throughout the day can help prevent symptoms such as bloating, reflux, and abdominal discomfort associated with gastrointestinal disorders. Additionally, avoiding large meals, especially before bedtime, can reduce the risk of symptoms such as heartburn and indigestion.

6. Mindful Eating: Practicing mindful eating techniques, such as chewing food slowly, avoiding distractions during meals, and paying attention to hunger and fullness cues, can help individuals with gastrointestinal disorders better manage their symptoms and improve digestion.

7. Seeking Professional Guidance: It's important for individuals with gastrointestinal disorders to work closely with healthcare providers, such as gastroenterologists and dietitians, to develop personalized diet and nutrition plans that address their specific needs, dietary restrictions, and symptom management goals. Professional guidance can help individuals navigate dietary challenges, ensure adequate nutrient intake, and optimize digestive health and overall well-being.

By incorporating these lifestyle modifications into their daily routines, individuals with gastrointestinal disorders can take proactive steps to manage their symptoms, improve digestive health, and enhance their quality of life.

Tips for meal planning and eating habits.

Tips for meal planning and eating habits for individuals with gastrointestinal disorders:

1. Identify Trigger Foods: Keep a food diary to track which foods exacerbate your symptoms. Common triggers include spicy foods, acidic foods, caffeine, alcohol, high-fat foods, gluten, and artificial sweeteners.

2. Focus on Whole Foods: Emphasize whole, minimally processed foods in your diet, such as fruits, vegetables, lean proteins, whole grains (if tolerated), nuts, seeds, and legumes.

3. Include Fiber-Rich Foods: Aim to incorporate fiber-rich foods, such as fruits, vegetables, whole grains, and legumes, to promote regular bowel movements and support digestive health. However, be mindful of fiber intake if you have certain conditions like Crohn's disease or diverticulitis.

4. Stay Hydrated: Drink plenty of water throughout the day to prevent dehydration and support digestion. Limit or avoid beverages that can exacerbate symptoms, such as caffeine, alcohol, and carbonated drinks.

5. Portion Control: Opt for smaller, more frequent meals and snacks to prevent overeating and reduce the risk of triggering symptoms like bloating and discomfort. Focus on portion control and listen to your body's hunger and fullness cues.

6. Meal Timing: Avoid eating large meals close to bedtime, as this can increase the risk of acid reflux and indigestion. Allow at least 2-3 hours between meals and bedtime to promote digestion and prevent nighttime symptoms.

7. Mindful Eating: Practice mindful eating by chewing food slowly, savoring each bite, and paying attention to hunger and fullness signals. Minimize distractions during meals, such as watching TV or using electronic devices.

The role of stress management and relaxation techniques.

Stress management and relaxation techniques play a crucial role in managing gastrointestinal disorders, as stress can exacerbate symptoms such as abdominal pain, bloating, diarrhea, and reflux. Here are some detailed techniques and how to practice them effectively:

1. Deep Breathing Exercises:
- Technique: Sit or lie down in a comfortable position. Close your eyes and take slow, deep breaths in through your nose, allowing your abdomen to expand. Hold the breath for a few seconds, then exhale slowly through your mouth, letting go of tension with each breath.
- How to do it: Practice deep breathing for 5-10 minutes daily, or whenever you feel stressed or anxious. You can use guided breathing apps or videos to help you focus and regulate your breath.

2. Progressive Muscle Relaxation (PMR):
- Technique: Start by tensing and then relaxing each muscle group in your body, one at a time, starting from your toes and working your way up to your head. Focus on the sensation of tension melting away as you release each muscle group.

- How to do it: Lie down in a comfortable position and close your eyes. Tense each muscle group for 5-10 seconds, then release and relax for 20-30 seconds before moving on to the next muscle group. Repeat the process for your entire body.

3. Mindfulness Meditation:
- Technique: Sit quietly and focus your attention on your breath, sensations in your body, or sounds around you. Notice any thoughts, feelings, or sensations that arise without judgment, and gently bring your attention back to your chosen focus.
- How to do it: Start with 5-10 minutes of mindfulness meditation daily, gradually increasing the duration as you become more comfortable. Use mindfulness apps or guided meditation recordings to help guide your practice.

4. Yoga:
- Technique: Practice gentle yoga poses, stretches, and breathing exercises to promote relaxation, improve flexibility, and reduce stress. Focus on connecting your breath with movement and being present in the moment.
- How to do it: Attend a yoga class led by a certified instructor, or follow along with online yoga videos or apps that cater to beginners or

individuals with specific health concerns, such as gastrointestinal disorders.

5. Guided Imagery:
- Technique: Close your eyes and visualize yourself in a peaceful, calming environment, such as a beach, forest, or garden. Engage all your senses by imagining the sights, sounds, smells, and sensations of that place.
- How to do it: Set aside 10-15 minutes in a quiet, comfortable space where you won't be disturbed. Use guided imagery scripts or recordings to guide your visualization and deepen your relaxation experience.

6. Journaling:
- Technique: Write down your thoughts, feelings, and experiences in a journal or notebook. Use journal prompts or free writing to explore your emotions, identify stressors, and reflect on positive aspects of your life.
- How to do it: Set aside a few minutes each day to journal, either in the morning to set intentions for the day ahead or in the evening to reflect on your day and unwind before bed.

Incorporate these stress management and relaxation techniques into your daily routine to help reduce stress, promote relaxation, and improve your overall well-being, including your digestive health. Experiment with different techniques to find what works best for you, and remember to be patient and consistent with your practice.

Chapter THREE: Specific Dietary Considerations

Overview of dietary modifications for each condition

Here's an overview of dietary modifications for each condition mentioned:

Gastro-Esophageal Reflux Disease (GERD):

- Dietary Modifications:
 - Avoid trigger foods such as spicy foods, acidic foods (citrus fruits, tomatoes), caffeine, alcohol, chocolate, and fatty or fried foods.
 - Eat smaller, more frequent meals to prevent overeating and reduce pressure on the lower esophageal sphincter (LES).
 - Avoid lying down or bending over immediately after eating. Allow at least 2-3 hours before lying down.
 - Elevate the head of the bed to reduce nighttime reflux symptoms.
 - Choose low-fat cooking methods and opt for lean proteins.
 - Increase fiber intake from fruits, vegetables, and whole grains to support digestion and prevent constipation.

Irritable Bowel Syndrome (IBS):

- Dietary Modifications:
  - Follow a low-FODMAP diet under the guidance of a healthcare provider or dietitian to identify and eliminate trigger foods high in fermentable carbohydrates.
  - Gradually reintroduce FODMAP foods to determine individual tolerance levels.
  - Increase fiber intake from soluble fiber sources such as oats, psyllium husk, and certain fruits and vegetables, while limiting insoluble fiber intake from foods like bran, beans, and raw vegetables.
  - Stay hydrated by drinking plenty of water throughout the day.
  - Avoid large meals and eat slowly to prevent overeating and reduce the risk of triggering symptoms.
  - Limit or avoid caffeine, alcohol, carbonated beverages, and artificial sweeteners, which can exacerbate symptoms in some individuals.

Gastritis:

- Dietary Modifications:
  - Avoid spicy foods, acidic foods (e.g., citrus fruits, tomatoes), caffeine, alcohol, and NSAIDs, which can irritate the stomach lining and exacerbate symptoms.

- Eat smaller, more frequent meals to reduce stomach acid production and minimize discomfort.
- Choose bland, easily digestible foods such as rice, bananas, applesauce, boiled potatoes, and lean proteins.
- Avoid eating close to bedtime to reduce the risk of acid reflux and nighttime symptoms.
- Incorporate probiotic-rich foods such as yogurt and kefir to promote a healthy balance of gut bacteria.
- Stay hydrated by drinking plenty of water, and consider drinking soothing herbal teas such as chamomile or ginger tea.

Celiac Disease:

- Dietary Modifications:
- Strictly adhere to a gluten-free diet, avoiding all sources of gluten including wheat, barley, rye, and cross-contaminated foods.
- Choose naturally gluten-free grains and flours such as rice, quinoa, corn, buckwheat, and certified gluten-free oats.
- Read food labels carefully and be aware of hidden sources of gluten in processed foods, sauces, condiments, and medications.
- Opt for whole, unprocessed foods and gluten-free alternatives to bread, pasta, and baked goods.

- Incorporate nutrient-dense foods such as fruits, vegetables, lean proteins, nuts, seeds, and legumes to ensure adequate nutrient intake.

Crohn's Disease:

- Dietary Modifications:
  - Experiment with a low-residue or low-fiber diet during flare-ups to reduce bowel movements and minimize irritation of the digestive tract.
  - Gradually reintroduce fiber-rich foods during remission to support digestive health and prevent constipation.
  - Stay hydrated by drinking plenty of water, and consider consuming electrolyte-rich beverages such as coconut water or sports drinks during periods of diarrhea or fluid loss.
  - Limit or avoid dairy products if lactose intolerance is a concern, and opt for lactose-free or dairy alternatives such as lactose-free milk or almond milk.
  - Monitor and limit intake of high-fat foods, spicy foods, caffeine, alcohol, and other potential trigger foods based on individual tolerance levels.
  - Consider working with a dietitian to develop a personalized nutrition plan that meets your specific needs and supports optimal digestive health.

Diverticulitis:

- Dietary Modifications:
  - During acute flare-ups, follow a clear liquid diet or low-fiber diet to rest the digestive tract and reduce inflammation. Gradually reintroduce low-fiber and then high-fiber foods as symptoms improve.
  - Increase fiber intake gradually to prevent constipation and promote regular bowel movements. Focus on soluble fiber sources such as oats, applesauce, bananas, and cooked vegetables.
  - Stay hydrated by drinking plenty of water and fluids throughout the day to soften stools and ease passage through the digestive tract.
  - Avoid foods that may exacerbate symptoms or irritate the digestive tract, such as nuts, seeds, popcorn, and tough or fibrous vegetables.
  - Monitor and limit intake of high-fat or fried foods, spicy foods, caffeine, and alcohol, which may worsen symptoms in some individuals.

Pancreatitis:

- Dietary Modifications:
  - Follow a low-fat diet to reduce strain on the pancreas and minimize the production of pancreatic enzymes. Limit or avoid fried

foods, fatty meats, full-fat dairy products, and high-fat desserts.
- Choose lean proteins such as poultry, fish, tofu, and legumes, and opt for cooking methods such as baking, steaming, boiling, or grilling instead of frying.
- Eat smaller, more frequent meals throughout the day to prevent overloading the pancreas and reduce the risk of triggering symptoms.
- Avoid or limit alcohol consumption, as it can exacerbate inflammation and increase the risk of pancreatitis flare-ups.
- Monitor blood sugar levels if pancreatitis has affected insulin production, and consider working with a dietitian to develop a balanced meal plan that supports blood sugar control and overall health.

By incorporating these specific dietary modifications into your lifestyle, you can better manage symptoms, reduce inflammation, and support optimal digestive health for each respective condition. Remember to consult with healthcare providers or registered dietitians for personalized dietary recommendations tailored to your individual needs and medical history.

Foods to avoid and foods to include(Recipes and Preparation Method Included)

Let's delve into specific foods to include and foods to avoid for each condition, along with recipes and preparation methods where applicable:

Gastro-Esophageal Reflux Disease (GERD):

Foods to Avoid:
- Spicy foods: Hot peppers, chili peppers, and spicy sauces.
- Acidic foods: Citrus fruits (e.g., oranges, lemons, grapefruits), tomatoes, and tomato-based products (e.g., pasta sauce, salsa).
- High-fat foods: Fried foods, fatty meats, full-fat dairy products (e.g., whole milk, cheese), and creamy sauces.
- Caffeine: Coffee, tea, chocolate, and caffeinated sodas.
- Alcohol: Beer, wine, and spirits.

Foods to Include:
- Lean proteins: Skinless poultry, fish, tofu, and legumes.

- Complex carbohydrates: Whole grains (e.g., brown rice, quinoa, oats), whole-wheat bread, and whole-grain pasta.
- Non-citrus fruits: Bananas, apples, melons, and pears.
- Vegetables: Leafy greens, broccoli, cauliflower, carrots, and green beans.
- Low-fat dairy alternatives: Skim milk, yogurt, and plant-based milk (e.g., almond milk).
- Herbal teas: Chamomile, ginger, and licorice root tea.

Recipe: Baked Herb-Crusted Salmon
- Ingredients: Salmon fillets, fresh herbs (e.g., parsley, dill, thyme), lemon zest, olive oil, salt, and pepper.
- Method:
   1. Preheat the oven to 375°F (190°C).
   2. In a small bowl, mix together chopped fresh herbs, lemon zest, olive oil, salt, and pepper to form a paste.
   3. Place the salmon fillets on a baking sheet lined with parchment paper.
   4. Spread the herb mixture evenly over the salmon fillets.
   5. Bake in the preheated oven for 12-15 minutes, or until the salmon is cooked through and flakes easily with a fork.
   6. Serve the herb-crusted salmon with steamed green beans and brown rice for a GERD-friendly meal.

Irritable Bowel Syndrome (IBS):

Foods to Avoid:
- High-FODMAP foods: Certain fruits (e.g., apples, cherries, watermelon), vegetables (e.g., onions, garlic, broccoli), legumes (e.g., beans, lentils), wheat products, and dairy products.
- Gas-producing foods: Carbonated beverages, cruciferous vegetables (e.g., cauliflower, cabbage, Brussels sprouts), and beans.
- High-fat foods: Fried foods, fatty meats, and creamy sauces.
- Caffeine: Coffee, tea, and caffeinated sodas.
- Artificial sweeteners: Sorbitol, mannitol, and xylitol found in sugar-free gum, candies, and beverages.

Foods to Include:
- Low-FODMAP fruits: Bananas, berries (e.g., strawberries, blueberries), grapes, and citrus fruits (in moderation).
- Low-FODMAP vegetables: Carrots, cucumber, zucchini, spinach, and bell peppers.
- Soluble fiber sources: Oats, psyllium husk, chia seeds, and flaxseeds.
- Lean proteins: Chicken, turkey, fish, tofu, and tempeh.

- Low-lactose dairy alternatives: Lactose-free milk, lactose-free yogurt, and aged cheeses (e.g., cheddar, Swiss).

Recipe: Quinoa Salad with Grilled Chicken
- Ingredients: Cooked quinoa, grilled chicken breast, diced cucumber, cherry tomatoes, chopped bell peppers, fresh parsley, lemon juice, olive oil, salt, and pepper.
- Method:
   1. In a large mixing bowl, combine cooked quinoa, diced grilled chicken breast, diced cucumber, halved cherry tomatoes, chopped bell peppers, and chopped fresh parsley.
   2. In a small bowl, whisk together lemon juice, olive oil, salt, and pepper to make the dressing.
   3. Pour the dressing over the quinoa salad and toss to coat evenly.
   4. Serve the quinoa salad chilled or at room temperature as a satisfying and IBS-friendly meal option.

Gastritis:

Foods to Avoid:
- Spicy foods: Hot peppers, chili peppers, and spicy sauces.
- Acidic foods: Citrus fruits (e.g., oranges, lemons, grapefruits), tomatoes, and tomato-based products (e.g., pasta sauce, salsa).

- High-fat foods: Fried foods, fatty meats, full-fat dairy products (e.g., whole milk, cheese), and creamy sauces.
- Caffeine: Coffee, tea, chocolate, and caffeinated sodas.
- Alcohol: Beer, wine, and spirits.

Foods to Include:
- Easily digestible foods: Boiled potatoes, plain rice, cooked oatmeal, and applesauce.
- Lean proteins: Baked or grilled chicken breast, turkey, fish, and tofu.
- Low-acid fruits: Bananas, melons (e.g., cantaloupe, honeydew), and apples (without skin).
- Cooked vegetables: Steamed or boiled carrots, green beans, squash, and spinach.
- Whole grains: White rice, white bread, and plain crackers.
- Herbal teas: Chamomile, ginger, and licorice root tea.

Recipe: Ginger

 Turmeric Chicken Soup
- Ingredients: Boneless, skinless chicken thighs or breasts, chicken broth, diced carrots, diced celery, diced onion, minced garlic, grated ginger, ground turmeric, salt, and pepper.
- Method:

1. In a large pot, heat olive oil over medium heat. Add diced onion, celery, and carrots, and sauté until softened.
2. Add minced garlic, grated ginger, and ground turmeric to the pot, and cook for another minute until fragrant.
3. Add chicken broth to the pot and bring to a simmer.
4. Add boneless, skinless chicken thighs or breasts to the pot, cover, and simmer until the chicken is cooked through and tender.
5. Remove the chicken from the pot and shred it using two forks. Return the shredded chicken to the pot.
6. Season the soup with salt and pepper to taste. Serve the ginger turmeric chicken soup hot as a soothing and gastritis-friendly meal option.

Celiac Disease:

Foods to Avoid:
- Gluten-containing grains: Wheat, barley, rye, and triticale.
- Processed foods: Bread, pasta, cereals, baked goods, and processed snacks containing gluten.
- Cross-contaminated foods: Foods prepared or processed in facilities that also handle gluten-containing ingredients.

- Sauces and condiments: Soy sauce, teriyaki sauce, and salad dressings containing wheat-based ingredients.
- Beer: Traditional beer made from barley malt.
- Some medications: Certain medications may contain gluten as a filler or binding agent.

Foods to Include:
- Naturally gluten-free grains: Rice, quinoa, corn, buckwheat, millet, and certified gluten-free oats.
- Gluten-free flours: Almond flour, coconut flour, chickpea flour, and gluten-free baking mixes.
- Fresh fruits and vegetables: Apples, bananas, berries, oranges, spinach, broccoli, carrots, and all other unprocessed fruits and vegetables.
- Lean proteins: Chicken, turkey, fish, eggs, tofu, and legumes.
- Dairy products: Milk, yogurt, cheese, and other lactose-free or dairy-free alternatives.
- Gluten-free snacks: Rice cakes, popcorn, nuts, seeds, and gluten-free crackers.

Recipe: Quinoa-Stuffed Bell Peppers
- Ingredients: Cooked quinoa, lean ground turkey or chicken, diced onion, diced bell peppers, minced garlic, diced tomatoes,

tomato sauce, shredded cheese (optional), salt, and pepper.
- Method:
  1. Preheat the oven to 375°F (190°C). Cut the tops off bell peppers and remove the seeds and membranes.
  2. In a skillet, cook lean ground turkey or chicken with diced onion, minced garlic, salt, and pepper until browned.
  3. Add cooked quinoa, diced tomatoes, and tomato sauce to the skillet, and stir to combine.
  4. Spoon the quinoa mixture into the hollowed-out bell peppers, and top with shredded cheese if desired.
  5. Place the stuffed bell peppers in a baking dish, cover with foil, and bake in the preheated oven for 30-35 minutes, or until the peppers are tender and the filling is heated through.
  6. Serve the quinoa-stuffed bell peppers as a nutritious and gluten-free meal option.

Crohn's Disease:

Foods to Avoid:
- High-fiber foods: Raw fruits and vegetables with skins, whole grains, nuts, seeds, and fibrous vegetables (e.g., broccoli, cauliflower).
- Gas-producing foods: Carbonated beverages, cruciferous vegetables (e.g.,

cabbage, Brussels sprouts), beans, and lentils.
- High-fat foods: Fried foods, fatty meats, creamy sauces, and rich desserts.
- Spicy foods: Hot peppers, chili peppers, and spicy sauces.
- Dairy products: Milk, cheese, and yogurt if lactose intolerant.
- Alcohol and caffeine: Beer, wine, spirits, coffee, tea, and caffeinated sodas.

Foods to Include:
- Low-fiber fruits and vegetables: Cooked or peeled fruits and vegetables, canned fruits (in juice), and well-cooked or pureed vegetables.
- Lean proteins: Chicken, turkey, fish, eggs, tofu, and smooth nut butters.
- Refined grains: White bread, white rice, refined pasta, and low-fiber cereals.
- Dairy alternatives: Lactose-free milk, lactose-free yogurt, and aged cheeses (e.g., cheddar, Swiss).
- Omega-3-rich foods: Fatty fish (e.g., salmon, mackerel), flaxseeds, chia seeds, and walnuts.
- Probiotic-rich foods: Yogurt with live active cultures, kefir, sauerkraut, and kimchi.

Recipe: Creamy Chicken and Rice Soup
- Ingredients: Cooked chicken breast, cooked white rice, diced carrots, diced celery, diced

onion, chicken broth, olive oil, minced garlic, dried thyme, salt, and pepper.
- Method:
   1. In a large pot, heat olive oil over medium heat. Add diced onion, celery, and carrots, and sauté until softened.
   2. Add minced garlic and dried thyme to the pot, and cook for another minute until fragrant.
   3. Add chicken broth to the pot and bring to a simmer.
   4. Add cooked chicken breast and cooked white rice to the pot, and simmer until heated through.
   5. Season the soup with salt and pepper to taste. Serve the creamy chicken and rice soup hot as a comforting and Crohn's-friendly meal option.

Diverticulitis:

Foods to Avoid:
- High-fiber foods: Raw fruits and vegetables with skins, whole grains, nuts, seeds, and fibrous vegetables (e.g., broccoli, cauliflower).
- Gas-producing foods: Carbonated beverages, cruciferous vegetables (e.g., cabbage, Brussels sprouts), beans, and lentils.
- Tough or fibrous meats: Tough cuts of meat, fatty meats, and processed meats (e.g., sausage, bacon).

- Spicy foods: Hot peppers, chili peppers, and spicy sauces.
- Alcohol and caffeine: Beer, wine, spirits, coffee, tea, and caffeinated sodas.
- High-fat foods: Fried foods, fatty meats, creamy sauces, and rich desserts.

Foods to Include:
- Low-fiber fruits and vegetables: Cooked or peeled fruits and vegetables, canned fruits (in juice), and well-cooked or pureed vegetables.
- Lean proteins: Chicken, turkey, fish, eggs, tofu, and smooth nut butters.
- Refined grains: White bread, white rice, refined pasta, and low-fiber cereals.
- Dairy alternatives: Lactose-free milk, lactose-free yogurt, and aged cheeses (e.g., cheddar, Swiss).
- Omega-3-rich foods: Fatty fish (e.g., salmon, mackerel), flaxseeds, chia seeds, and walnuts.
- Probiotic-rich foods: Yogurt with live active cultures, kefir, sauerkraut, and kimchi.

Recipe: Mashed Sweet Potatoes
- Ingredients: Sweet potatoes, unsweetened almond milk (or lactose-free milk), olive oil, salt, and pepper.
- Method:

1. Peel and chop sweet potatoes into chunks.
2. Place the sweet potato chunks in a pot of water and bring to a boil. Cook until the sweet potatoes are fork-tender.
3. Drain the cooked sweet potatoes and transfer them to a mixing bowl.
4. Add unsweetened almond milk (or lactose-free milk), olive oil, salt, and pepper to taste.
5. Mash the sweet potatoes using a potato masher or fork until smooth and creamy.
6. Serve the mashed sweet potatoes as a delicious and diverticulitis-friendly side dish.

Pancreatitis:

Foods to Avoid:
- High-fat foods: Fried foods, fatty meats, full-fat dairy products (e.g., whole milk, cheese), and creamy sauces.
- Spicy foods: Hot peppers, chili peppers, and spicy sauces.
- Alcohol: Beer, wine, and spirits.
- Caffeine: Coffee, tea, chocolate, and caffeinated sodas.
- Sugary foods: Sweets, pastries, and desserts high in added sugars.
- Processed foods: Processed snacks, fast food, and packaged meals high in trans fats and artificial additives.

Foods to Include:
- Lean proteins: Skinless poultry, fish, tofu, and legumes.
- Low-fat dairy alternatives: Skim milk, yogurt, and plant-based milk (e.g., almond milk).
- Whole grains: Brown rice, quinoa, whole-wheat bread (in moderation), and whole-grain pasta.
- Cooked or steamed vegetables: Carrots, green beans, squash, and spinach.
- Non-citrus fruits: Bananas, melons, and applesauce.
- Herbal teas: Chamomile, ginger, and licorice root tea.

Recipe: Baked Chicken and Vegetables
- Ingredients: Chicken breasts, diced carrots, diced zucchini, diced bell peppers, minced garlic, olive oil, dried herbs (e.g., thyme, rosemary), salt, and pepper.
- Method:
  1. Preheat the oven to 375°F (190°C). Place chicken breasts in a baking dish.
  2. In a mixing bowl, toss diced carrots, diced zucchini, diced bell peppers, minced garlic, olive oil, dried herbs, salt, and pepper until evenly coated.
  3. Arrange the seasoned vegetables around the chicken breasts in the baking dish.

4. Bake in the preheated oven for 25-30 minutes, or until the chicken is cooked through and the vegetables are tender.

5. Serve the baked chicken and vegetables as a wholesome and pancreatitis-friendly meal option.

These specific dietary recommendations, along with the provided recipes and preparation methods, can help individuals with gastrointestinal disorders navigate their dietary choices and optimize their nutrition while managing their condition. It's important to consult with healthcare providers or registered dietitians for personalized dietary advice tailored to individual needs, preferences, and medical history.

General Meal ideas and recipes tailored to accommodate every GI disease mentioned

Certainly! Here are some general meal ideas and recipes tailored to accommodate individuals with gastrointestinal diseases mentioned, including GERD, IBS, gastritis, celiac disease, Crohn's disease, diverticulitis, and pancreatitis:

Breakfast Ideas:

1. Oatmeal with Banana and Almond Butter:
   - Cooked oats topped with sliced banana, a dollop of almond butter, and a sprinkle of cinnamon. Serve with a side of lactose-free yogurt or almond milk.

2. Scrambled Tofu with Spinach and Tomatoes:
   - Scrambled tofu cooked with sautéed spinach, cherry tomatoes, and minced garlic. Season with turmeric, salt, and pepper. Serve with a slice of gluten-free toast.

3. Smoothie Bowl:
   - Blend together frozen mixed berries, spinach, banana, almond milk, and a scoop of protein powder. Top with gluten-free granola, sliced almonds, and fresh berries.

Lunch Ideas:

1. Quinoa Salad with Grilled Chicken:
   - Cooked quinoa mixed with diced cucumber, cherry tomatoes, bell peppers, and chopped parsley. Toss with lemon-tahini dressing and top with grilled chicken breast slices.

2. Baked Salmon with Steamed Vegetables:
   - Baked salmon seasoned with lemon zest, dill, and garlic. Serve with steamed carrots, green beans, and squash. Accompany with a side of mashed sweet potatoes.

3. Turkey and Avocado Wrap:
   - Gluten-free tortilla filled with sliced turkey breast, mashed avocado, lettuce, tomato, and cucumber. Serve with a side of carrot sticks and hummus.

Dinner Ideas:

1. Stir-Fried Tofu with Mixed Vegetables:
   - Cubed tofu stir-fried with broccoli, bell peppers, snap peas, carrots, and mushrooms in a ginger-soy sauce. Serve over brown rice or quinoa.

2. Chicken and Vegetable Curry:
   - Chicken breast simmered in a coconut milk-based curry sauce with onions, garlic, ginger, and mixed vegetables (e.g., cauliflower, peas, carrots). Serve with basmati rice or cauliflower rice.

3. Grilled Shrimp Skewers with Quinoa Salad:
   - Marinated shrimp skewers grilled with cherry tomatoes, zucchini, and red onion.

Serve with a quinoa salad mixed with diced cucumber, mint, feta cheese, and lemon vinaigrette.

Snack Ideas:

1. Rice Cake with Almond Butter and Banana Slices:
   - Brown rice cake topped with almond butter and thinly sliced banana. Sprinkle with chia seeds for added crunch.

2. Greek Yogurt Parfait with Berries and Granola:
   - Layer lactose-free Greek yogurt with fresh berries and gluten-free granola in a glass. Repeat layers and drizzle with honey.

3. Trail Mix:
   - Mix together unsalted nuts (e.g., almonds, walnuts), seeds (e.g., pumpkin seeds, sunflower seeds), and dried fruits (e.g., raisins, apricots) for a portable and nutritious snack.

Dessert Ideas:

1. Baked Apples with Cinnamon and Walnuts:

- Core apples and fill with a mixture of chopped walnuts, cinnamon, and a drizzle of honey. Bake until tender and serve warm.

2. Dark Chocolate Covered Strawberries:
   - Dip fresh strawberries in melted dark chocolate and place on a parchment-lined baking sheet. Allow to set in the refrigerator before serving.

3. Coconut Chia Pudding:
   - Mix together coconut milk, chia seeds, and a touch of maple syrup. Let it sit in the refrigerator overnight to thicken. Serve topped with fresh berries.

These meal ideas and recipes are designed to accommodate individuals with various gastrointestinal diseases by incorporating ingredients and cooking methods that are gentle on the digestive system and align with dietary restrictions specific to each condition. Adjustments can be made based on individual preferences, tolerances, and nutritional needs. It's advisable to consult with healthcare providers or registered dietitians for personalized dietary recommendations tailored to individual health concerns and goals.

Chapter FOUR: Medications and Supplements:

Overview of common medications prescribed for each gastrointestinal disorders

Here's an overview of common medications prescribed for each gastrointestinal disorder mentioned:

Gastro-Esophageal Reflux Disease (GERD):

1. Proton Pump Inhibitors (PPIs):
   - Examples: Omeprazole (Prilosec), Esomeprazole (Nexium), Lansoprazole (Prevacid).
   - Mechanism: Reduce stomach acid production by blocking the proton pump in the stomach lining.
   - Indication: Treatment of frequent heartburn, acid reflux, and GERD symptoms.

2. H2 Receptor Antagonists:

- Examples: Ranitidine (Zantac), Famotidine (Pepcid), Cimetidine (Tagamet).
- Mechanism: Reduce stomach acid production by blocking histamine receptors in the stomach lining.
- Indication: Relief of mild to moderate heartburn, acid indigestion, and GERD symptoms.

3. Antacids:
- Examples: Tums, Rolaids, Maalox, Mylanta.
- Mechanism: Neutralize stomach acid and provide rapid but short-term relief of heartburn and acid reflux symptoms.
- Indication: On-demand relief of occasional heartburn and indigestion.

Irritable Bowel Syndrome (IBS):

1. Antispasmodics:
- Examples: Dicyclomine (Bentyl), Hyoscyamine (Levsin), Peppermint oil.
- Mechanism: Relieve abdominal cramping and spasms by relaxing smooth muscles in the digestive tract.
- Indication: Alleviation of abdominal pain and discomfort associated with IBS.

2. Fiber Supplements:

- Examples: Psyllium husk (Metamucil), Methylcellulose (Citrucel), Polycarbophil (FiberCon).
   - Mechanism: Increase stool bulk and improve bowel regularity by providing soluble fiber.
   - Indication: Management of constipation-predominant IBS symptoms.

3. Probiotics:
   - Examples: Lactobacillus, Bifidobacterium, Saccharomyces boulardii.
   - Mechanism: Restore and maintain a healthy balance of gut bacteria, which may help alleviate IBS symptoms.
   - Indication: Reduction of bloating, gas, and abdominal discomfort in some individuals with IBS.

Gastritis:

1. Proton Pump Inhibitors (PPIs):
   - Examples: Omeprazole (Prilosec), Esomeprazole (Nexium), Lansoprazole (Prevacid).
   - Mechanism: Suppress stomach acid production to promote healing of the gastric mucosa and alleviate gastritis symptoms.

- Indication: Treatment of gastritis, peptic ulcers, and Gastro-Esophageal Reflux disease (GERD).

2. Antibiotics:
   - Examples: Clarithromycin, Amoxicillin, Metronidazole.
   - Mechanism: Eradicate Helicobacter pylori bacteria, a common cause of chronic gastritis and peptic ulcers.
   - Indication: Combination therapy with PPIs for H. pylori-associated gastritis and peptic ulcer disease.

3. Antacids and H2 Receptor Antagonists:
   - Examples: Aluminum hydroxide, Calcium carbonate, Ranitidine (Zantac), Famotidine (Pepcid).
   - Mechanism: Neutralize stomach acid or reduce its production to provide symptomatic relief of gastritis.

Celiac Disease:

1. Gluten-Free Diet:
   - Mechanism: Strict avoidance of gluten-containing foods and ingredients to prevent intestinal damage and autoimmune response.

- Indication: Essential lifelong treatment for individuals with celiac disease to manage symptoms and prevent complications.

2. Vitamin and Mineral Supplements:
   - Examples: Iron, Calcium, Vitamin D, Vitamin B12, Folate.
   - Mechanism: Address nutritional deficiencies commonly associated with malabsorption and intestinal damage in celiac disease.
   - Indication: Support optimal nutrient intake and prevent or treat deficiencies due to gluten-related damage to the small intestine.

Crohn's Disease:

1. Anti-Inflammatory Medications:
   - Examples: Mesalamine (Asacol, Pentasa), Sulfasalazine (Azulfidine).
   - Mechanism: Reduce inflammation in the digestive tract and help control mild to moderate Crohn's disease symptoms.
   - Indication: Maintenance therapy to prevent flare-ups and promote remission in patients with mild to moderate disease activity.

2. Immunosuppressants:
   - Examples: Azathioprine (Imuran), Mercaptopurine (Purinethol), Methotrexate.

- Mechanism: Suppress the immune system to reduce inflammation and prevent immune-mediated damage to the intestinal lining.
- Indication: Treatment of moderate to severe Crohn's disease that is unresponsive to other medications or requires long-term management.

3. Biologic Therapies:
- Examples: Infliximab (Remicade), Adalimumab (Humira), Vedolizumab (Entyvio).
- Mechanism: Target specific proteins involved in the inflammatory response to reduce inflammation and induce remission.
- Indication: Treatment of moderate to severe Crohn's disease that is refractory to conventional therapies or requires rapid control of symptoms.

Diverticulitis:

1. Antibiotics:
- Examples: Ciprofloxacin, Metronidazole, Amoxicillin-clavulanate.
- Mechanism: Eradicate bacterial infection and reduce inflammation in the diverticula of the colon during acute episodes of diverticulitis.

   - Indication: Short-term antibiotic therapy for uncomplicated diverticulitis or as part of combination therapy for complicated cases.

2. Pain Relievers:
   - Examples: Acetaminophen, Ibuprofen (in some cases).
   - Mechanism: Provide relief from abdominal pain and discomfort associated with diverticulitis.
   - Indication: Symptomatic treatment of

 mild to moderate pain during acute episodes of diverticulitis.

Pancreatitis:

1. Pain Management:
   - Examples: Acetaminophen, Nonsteroidal anti-inflammatory drugs (NSAIDs).
   - Mechanism: Alleviate abdominal pain and discomfort associated with acute pancreatitis.
   - Indication: Symptomatic relief of mild to moderate pain during acute episodes of pancreatitis.

2. Pancreatic Enzyme Replacement Therapy (PERT):
   - Examples: Pancrelipase (Creon, Pancreaze), Pancreatin (Pangestyme).

- Mechanism: Supplement pancreatic enzymes to aid digestion and improve nutrient absorption in individuals with pancreatic insufficiency.
- Indication: Long-term management of chronic pancreatitis and exocrine pancreatic insufficiency.

3. Intravenous Fluids and Nutrition:
- Mechanism: Provide hydration, electrolyte balance, and essential nutrients through intravenous fluids and total parenteral nutrition (TPN) during acute pancreatitis episodes with severe symptoms or complications.

It's important for individuals with gastrointestinal disorders to follow their healthcare provider's recommendations regarding medication use, dosage, and duration of treatment. Additionally, regular monitoring and follow-up appointments are essential to assess treatment effectiveness, manage potential side effects, and make adjustments to the treatment plan as needed.

Potential side effects and interactions

Here's an overview of potential side effects and interactions associated with common medications used to treat gastrointestinal disorders:

Gastro-Esophageal Reflux Disease (GERD):

1. Proton Pump Inhibitors (PPIs):
  - Side Effects: Headache, diarrhea, abdominal pain, nausea, and increased risk of bone fractures with long-term use.
  - Interactions: Decreased absorption of certain medications (e.g., iron supplements, anti-fungal drugs), increased risk of Clostridium difficile infection, and potential interactions with antiplatelet and anticoagulant medications.

2. H2 Receptor Antagonists:
  - Side Effects: Headache, dizziness, diarrhea, constipation, and potential for vitamin B12 deficiency with long-term use.
  - Interactions: Reduced absorption of certain medications (e.g., antifungal drugs, calcium channel blockers), increased risk of Clostridium difficile infection, and potential interactions with antiplatelet and anticoagulant medications.

3. Antacids:

- Side Effects: Constipation or diarrhea, electrolyte imbalances (with excessive use), and potential for drug interactions (e.g., reduced absorption of certain medications such as antibiotics, thyroid medications).
- Interactions: Reduced absorption of certain medications (e.g., tetracycline antibiotics, fluoroquinolone antibiotics, iron supplements), and potential interactions with other medications taken simultaneously.

Irritable Bowel Syndrome (IBS):

1. Antispasmodics:
- Side Effects: Dry mouth, blurred vision, dizziness, constipation, and urinary retention.
- Interactions: Potential interactions with medications that affect heart rate and blood pressure (e.g., beta-blockers, calcium channel blockers), and increased sedation when used concomitantly with other central nervous system depressants.

2. Fiber Supplements:
- Side Effects: Flatulence, bloating, abdominal discomfort, and potential for bowel obstruction or impaction if not taken with adequate fluids.
- Interactions: Reduced absorption of certain medications (e.g., digoxin, warfarin), and

potential interactions with other medications taken simultaneously.

3. Probiotics:
   - Side Effects: Gas, bloating, and abdominal discomfort, especially during the initial period of use.
   - Interactions: Potential interactions with immunosuppressive medications, antibiotics, and antifungal drugs, and caution advised in individuals with compromised immune function or underlying health conditions.

Gastritis:

1. Proton Pump Inhibitors (PPIs):
   - Side Effects: Headache, diarrhea, abdominal pain, nausea, and increased risk of bone fractures with long-term use.
   - Interactions: Decreased absorption of certain medications (e.g., iron supplements, anti-fungal drugs), increased risk of Clostridium difficile infection, and potential interactions with antiplatelet and anticoagulant medications.

2. Antibiotics:
   - Side Effects: Nausea, vomiting, diarrhea, abdominal pain, and potential for allergic reactions or adverse effects on liver function.

- Interactions: Potential interactions with other medications metabolized by the liver, and caution advised in individuals with known allergies or sensitivities to antibiotics.

3. Antacids and H2 Receptor Antagonists:
   - Side Effects: Similar to those mentioned in the GERD section.
   - Interactions: Similar to those mentioned in the GERD section.

Celiac Disease:

1. Gluten-Free Diet:
   - Side Effects: None specific to the diet itself, but adherence to a strict gluten-free diet may pose challenges in social situations, dining out, and food preparation.
   - Interactions: None related to medication interactions, but caution advised in ensuring strict adherence to a gluten-free diet to prevent symptoms and complications associated with celiac disease.

2. Vitamin and Mineral Supplements:
   - Side Effects: Generally well-tolerated when taken as directed, but potential for gastrointestinal upset, constipation, or diarrhea with high doses.

- Interactions: Potential interactions with certain medications (e.g., iron supplements may decrease absorption of certain antibiotics), and caution advised in individuals with underlying health conditions or predisposing factors.

Crohn's Disease:

1. Anti-Inflammatory Medications:
  - Side Effects: Nausea, vomiting, diarrhea, abdominal pain, headache, and potential for adverse effects on liver function or blood cell counts with long-term use.
  - Interactions: Potential interactions with other medications metabolized by the liver, and caution advised in individuals with known allergies or sensitivities to anti-inflammatory drugs.

2. Immunosuppressants:
  - Side Effects: Increased risk of infections, bone marrow suppression, liver toxicity, and potential for allergic reactions or infusion-related reactions.
  - Interactions: Potential interactions with other immunosuppressive medications, and caution advised in individuals with compromised immune function or underlying health conditions.

3. Biologic Therapies:
  - Side Effects: Injection site reactions, infusion-related reactions, increased risk of infections, and potential for allergic reactions.
  - Interactions: Potential interactions with other immunosuppressive medications, and caution advised in individuals with compromised immune function or underlying health conditions.

Diverticulitis:

1. Antibiotics:
  - Side Effects: Similar to those mentioned in the Gastritis section.
  - Interactions: Similar to those mentioned in the Gastritis section.

2. Pain Relievers:
  - Side Effects: Similar to those mentioned in the Crohn's Disease section.
  - Interactions: Similar to those mentioned in the Crohn's Disease section.

Pancreatitis:

1. Pain Management:
  - Side Effects: Similar to those mentioned in the Crohn's Disease section.

- Interactions: Similar to those mentioned in the Crohn's Disease section.

2. Pancreatic Enzyme Replacement Therapy (PERT):
   - Side Effects: Gastrointestinal upset, abdominal pain, diarrhea, and potential for allergic reactions.
   - Interactions: Potential interactions with other medications metabolized by the liver or affected by changes in gastrointestinal pH.

It's important for individuals to be aware of potential side effects and interactions associated with medications used to treat gastrointestinal disorders and to discuss any concerns with their healthcare provider. Additionally, healthcare providers should be informed of all medications, supplements, and over-the-counter products being used to prevent potential interactions and adverse effects. Regular monitoring and follow-up appointments are essential to ensure safe and effective treatment management.

Role of supplements in managing symptoms (Including highly trusted supplements and how to get them).

Supplements can play a supportive role in managing symptoms of gastrointestinal disorders by addressing specific nutritional deficiencies, promoting gut health, and alleviating digestive discomfort. Here's an overview of some commonly used supplements and their roles in managing symptoms:

Probiotics:

Role: Probiotics are beneficial bacteria that help maintain a healthy balance of gut microbiota, support digestion, and strengthen the immune system. They may also help alleviate symptoms such as bloating, gas, and diarrhea, especially in conditions like IBS and certain types of gastritis.

Highly Trusted Supplements:
- Culturelle Digestive Health Probiotic: Contains Lactobacillus rhamnosus GG, a well-studied probiotic strain known for its digestive health benefits.
- Align Probiotic Supplement: Contains Bifidobacterium infantis 35624, which has

been clinically shown to support digestive balance.
- Florastor Daily Probiotic Supplement: Contains Saccharomyces boulardii, a beneficial yeast strain that helps maintain intestinal health and supports immune function.

How to Get Them: Probiotic supplements are widely available over-the-counter at pharmacies, health food stores, and online retailers. Look for supplements that contain well-researched strains, are third-party tested for quality and potency, and have positive customer reviews. It's important to follow the recommended dosage instructions provided on the product label or as directed by a healthcare professional.

Digestive Enzymes:

Role: Digestive enzymes help break down macronutrients (carbohydrates, proteins, and fats) into smaller molecules for better absorption and digestion. They can be especially beneficial for individuals with conditions like pancreatic insufficiency, celiac disease, and certain types of gastritis where enzyme production may be impaired.

Highly Trusted Supplements:

- NOW Super Enzymes: A comprehensive blend of enzymes including amylase, protease, lipase, cellulase, and more to support healthy digestion.
- Enzymedica Digest Gold: Contains a potent blend of digestive enzymes, including specialized enzymes for gluten and dairy digestion, to assist with nutrient absorption and reduce digestive discomfort.
- Garden of Life Organic Digest+: Formulated with organic whole foods and digestive enzymes to support optimal digestion and nutrient absorption.

How to Get Them: Digestive enzyme supplements are available in capsule, tablet, and powder forms and can be purchased over-the-counter at pharmacies, health food stores, and online retailers. Look for supplements that contain a broad spectrum of enzymes and are specifically formulated to address your digestive needs. It's advisable to consult with a healthcare professional before starting enzyme supplementation, especially if you have underlying health conditions or are taking medications.

Fish Oil/Omega-3 Fatty Acids:

Role: Omega-3 fatty acids, particularly EPA (eicosapentaenoic acid) and DHA (docosahexaenoic acid) found in fish oil, have anti-inflammatory properties and may help reduce inflammation in conditions like Crohn's disease and ulcerative colitis. They may also support heart health and overall well-being.

Highly Trusted Supplements:
- Nordic Naturals Ultimate Omega: A high-potency fish oil supplement with concentrated levels of EPA and DHA to support cardiovascular health and reduce inflammation.
- Carlson Labs Elite Omega-3 Gems: Molecularly distilled fish oil capsules with high levels of omega-3 fatty acids and lemon-flavored enteric coating for improved absorption and reduced fishy aftertaste.
- NOW Ultra Omega-3: A softgel formulation containing fish oil derived from sustainably sourced fish and providing optimal levels of EPA and DHA for overall health support.

How to Get Them: Fish oil supplements are available in liquid and softgel formulations and can be purchased over-the-counter at pharmacies, health food stores, and online retailers. Look for supplements that are molecularly distilled to remove impurities and meet quality standards. It's important to choose fish oil supplements from reputable brands that adhere to sustainable fishing practices and offer third-party testing for purity and potency.

When selecting supplements for managing gastrointestinal symptoms, it's essential to consult with a healthcare professional, such as a registered dietitian or gastroenterologist, to determine the appropriate type, dosage, and duration of supplementation based on individual health needs and conditions. Additionally, it's important to follow the recommended usage instructions provided by the supplement manufacturer and to monitor for any adverse reactions or interactions with other medications or supplements.

Chapter FIVE: Coping Strategies and Emotional Support

Dealing with the emotional impact of living with a chronic digestive condition

Living with a chronic digestive condition can be emotionally challenging, often causing feelings of frustration, anxiety, and even depression. It's completely normal to experience a range of emotions when navigating the ups and downs of managing your health. Remember, you're not alone in this journey, and there are coping strategies and sources of emotional support that can help you navigate these challenges:

1. Seek Support from Loved Ones: Don't hesitate to lean on friends, family members, or support groups for emotional support. Sharing your experiences and feelings with trusted individuals can provide comfort and understanding.

2. Educate Yourself: Knowledge is empowering. Take the time to educate yourself about your condition, treatment options, and lifestyle modifications. Understanding your condition better can help you feel more in control and confident in managing it.

3. Practice Self-Compassion: Be kind to yourself and acknowledge that living with a chronic condition is not easy. Allow yourself to feel your emotions without judgment and practice self-care activities that bring you comfort and relaxation.

4. Stay Connected: Stay connected with others who understand what you're going through, whether it's through online support groups, forums, or local support networks. Sharing experiences with others who can relate can provide a sense of validation and community.

5. Communicate with Healthcare Providers: Open and honest communication with your healthcare providers is key. Don't hesitate to discuss any concerns or emotional struggles you're experiencing. They can offer guidance, support, and resources to help you cope effectively.

6. Engage in Stress-Relief Activities: Explore stress-relief techniques such as mindfulness meditation, deep breathing exercises, yoga, or tai chi. These practices can help reduce stress, promote relaxation, and improve overall well-being.

7. Focus on What You Can Control: While you may not be able to control your condition entirely, focus on the aspects of your life that you can control, such as your diet, lifestyle habits, and self-care routines. Small changes can make a big difference in how you feel physically and emotionally.

8. Set Realistic Goals: Set achievable goals for yourself and celebrate your progress along the way. Breaking larger goals into smaller, manageable steps can make them feel more attainable and boost your confidence.

9. Stay Positive: Maintain a positive outlook and focus on the things in your life that bring you joy and fulfillment. Even on difficult days, try to find moments of gratitude and optimism.

10. Seek Professional Help if Needed: If you're struggling to cope with the emotional impact of your condition, don't hesitate to seek professional help from a therapist, counselor, or psychologist. They can provide valuable

support, coping strategies, and tools to help you navigate your emotions more effectively.

Remember, it's okay to have good days and bad days, and it's okay to ask for help when you need it. You're stronger than you realize, and with the right support and coping strategies, you can navigate the emotional challenges of living with a chronic digestive condition with resilience and grace.

Support networks and resources available for patients and caregivers

Navigating life with a chronic digestive condition can feel overwhelming at times, but there are numerous support networks and resources available to provide assistance and guidance to both patients and caregivers:

1. Patient Advocacy Organizations: Organizations such as the Crohn's & Colitis Foundation, the American Gastroenterological Association (AGA), the International Foundation for Gastrointestinal Disorders (IFFGD), and the Celiac Disease Foundation offer a wealth of resources, including educational materials, support groups, online forums, and advocacy initiatives.

2. Online Support Communities: Websites and online forums like Inspire, PatientsLikeMe, and HealingWell provide platforms for patients and caregivers to connect with others facing similar challenges, share experiences, ask questions, and offer support in a safe and understanding environment.

3. Local Support Groups: Many communities have local support groups or chapters affiliated with larger advocacy organizations. These groups often meet in person or virtually to provide peer support, education, and resources specific to the needs of individuals living with digestive conditions and their caregivers.

4. Educational Workshops and Webinars: Patient advocacy organizations and healthcare institutions frequently host educational workshops, webinars, and conferences focused on various digestive conditions. These events cover topics such as treatment options, symptom management, nutrition, and coping strategies.

5. Telehealth Services: Telehealth platforms and virtual healthcare providers offer convenient access to healthcare professionals, including gastroenterologists,

dietitians, psychologists, and counselors. Patients and caregivers can schedule virtual appointments, receive medical advice, and access specialized care from the comfort of their own homes.

6. Caregiver Support Resources: Caregivers play a crucial role in supporting individuals with chronic digestive conditions. Resources such as caregiver support groups, online forums, and educational materials provide caregivers with information, validation, and practical tips for managing their caregiving responsibilities while prioritizing their own well-being.

7. Educational Materials and Publications: Patient advocacy organizations, healthcare institutions, and reputable medical websites publish a variety of educational materials, brochures, fact sheets, and newsletters covering topics related to digestive health. These resources offer reliable information and practical guidance for patients and caregivers alike.

8. Social Media Communities: Social media platforms like Facebook, Twitter, and Instagram host numerous communities and pages dedicated to digestive health advocacy, patient support, and awareness campaigns.

Patients and caregivers can connect with like-minded individuals, share resources, and participate in online events and discussions.

9. Hospital and Clinic Programs: Many hospitals and healthcare facilities offer specialized programs and services for patients with digestive conditions, including multidisciplinary care teams, nutrition counseling, psychosocial support services, and integrative therapies such as acupuncture and mindfulness meditation.

10. Government Health Agencies: Government agencies such as the National Institutes of Health (NIH), the Centers for Disease Control and Prevention (CDC), and the Food and Drug Administration (FDA) provide valuable information, research updates, and resources related to digestive health, treatment options, and patient safety.

By tapping into these support networks and resources, patients and caregivers can access valuable information, connect with others facing similar challenges, and gain the support, encouragement, and guidance needed to navigate the journey of living with a chronic digestive condition with resilience and empowerment.

Chapter SIX: Practical Tips for Everyday Living:

Living with a chronic digestive condition requires thoughtful planning and strategies to manage symptoms effectively, both at home and on the go. Here are some practical tips for everyday living to help individuals cope with their condition:

Managing Symptoms at Home:

1. Maintain a Symptom Journal: Keep track of your symptoms, triggers, and dietary intake in a journal or mobile app. This can help identify patterns and make informed decisions about managing your condition.

2. Follow a Consistent Meal Schedule: Eat regular, smaller meals throughout the day to avoid overloading your digestive system. Stick to a balanced diet rich in fiber, fruits, vegetables, lean proteins, and healthy fats.

3. Stay Hydrated: Drink plenty of water throughout the day to help maintain hydration and support digestion. Limit intake of

caffeinated and alcoholic beverages, as they can exacerbate symptoms.

4. Practice Stress Management: Engage in relaxation techniques such as deep breathing, meditation, yoga, or tai chi to reduce stress and promote overall well-being. Stress can exacerbate digestive symptoms, so finding ways to manage stress is essential.

5. Get Adequate Sleep: Prioritize quality sleep by establishing a regular sleep schedule, creating a calming bedtime routine, and optimizing your sleep environment. Sufficient sleep is crucial for overall health and can help manage symptoms.

6. Incorporate Physical Activity: Stay active with regular exercise tailored to your abilities and preferences. Aim for at least 30 minutes of moderate-intensity exercise most days of the week to support digestion and reduce stress.

7. Practice Good Hygiene: Wash your hands regularly, especially before handling food or eating, to reduce the risk of gastrointestinal infections. Follow proper food safety guidelines when preparing and storing food.

8. Stock Up on Digestive Comfort Aids: Keep over-the-counter medications, such as antacids, anti-diarrheal agents, and pain relievers, on hand to manage acute symptoms as needed. Consult your healthcare provider for guidance on appropriate use.

Managing Symptoms On the Go:

1. Pack Portable Snacks: Carry easily digestible snacks such as rice cakes, bananas, crackers, or trail mix to have on hand when hunger strikes or as a buffer between meals.

2. Plan Ahead for Meals: Research restaurant menus in advance, choose eateries with options that align with your dietary needs, and communicate your preferences to waitstaff to ensure a comfortable dining experience.

3. Bring Water Everywhere: Carry a refillable water bottle with you wherever you go to stay hydrated throughout the day. Opt for plain water or infused water with lemon or cucumber for added flavor.

4. Know Restroom Locations: Familiarize yourself with restroom locations in public spaces and plan your outings accordingly,

especially if you experience urgency or frequent bathroom trips.

5. Pack a Symptom Relief Kit: Prepare a small kit containing essentials such as hand sanitizer, wet wipes, tissues, and any medications or supplements you may need to manage symptoms while away from home.

6. Practice Mindful Eating: Take your time to chew food thoroughly, eat slowly, and pay attention to your body's hunger and fullness cues. Avoid rushing meals or overeating, as this can exacerbate digestive discomfort.

7. Listen to Your Body: Honor your body's signals and prioritize self-care. If you're feeling fatigued or experiencing flare-ups, don't hesitate to take breaks, rest when needed, and adjust your activities accordingly.

By incorporating these practical tips into your daily routine, you can better manage symptoms, minimize discomfort, and maintain a sense of control over your digestive condition, both at home and on the go. Remember to consult with your healthcare provider for personalized guidance and support tailored to your individual needs and condition.

Traveling with dietary restrictions

Traveling with dietary restrictions can present unique challenges, but with careful planning and preparation, it's possible to enjoy fulfilling and stress-free travel experiences. Here are some insights and tips for navigating travel with dietary restrictions:

Before You Go:

1. Research Destination: Before traveling, research your destination's food options, local cuisine, and availability of dietary-friendly restaurants or grocery stores. Look for online resources, travel guides, and forums where fellow travelers share their experiences and recommendations.

2. Plan Meals and Snacks: Identify restaurants, cafes, or grocery stores that offer options aligned with your dietary needs. Consider packing portable snacks and meal alternatives, such as protein bars, nuts, dried fruits, and gluten-free crackers, to have on hand during travel days or outings.

3. Communicate Dietary Needs: Inform airlines, hotels, tour operators, and restaurants about your dietary restrictions in advance. Many establishments are willing to

accommodate special requests with advance notice, so don't hesitate to communicate your needs clearly and politely.

4. Pack Essentials: Pack essential items such as non-perishable snacks, dietary supplements, and medications in your carry-on luggage to ensure you have access to them during transit. Consider bringing a small cooler bag or insulated container for perishable items.

During Your Trip:

1. Read Labels and Menus: When dining out or shopping for food, carefully read ingredient labels and menu descriptions to identify potential allergens or ingredients that may not be suitable for your dietary restrictions. Ask questions or seek clarification from restaurant staff if needed.

2. Choose Safe Options: Opt for simple, minimally processed foods and dishes that are naturally free of your allergens or dietary triggers. Choose customizable options or dishes that can be modified to meet your needs, such as salads without croutons or dressings on the side.

3. Be Prepared for Language Barriers: If traveling to a foreign country where you may encounter language barriers, consider learning key phrases or terms related to your dietary restrictions. Carry a printed or digital card explaining your dietary needs in the local language to facilitate communication with locals and restaurant staff.

4. Explore Local Markets: Visit local markets, farmers' markets, or specialty food stores to discover fresh, locally sourced ingredients and specialty products that align with your dietary preferences. Engage with vendors to learn about traditional dishes and ingredients that may be suitable for your restrictions.

5. BYOF (Bring Your Own Food): For added peace of mind, consider bringing a selection of your own pre-prepared meals, snacks, or ingredients that you know are safe and suitable for your dietary needs. This can be particularly helpful during long flights, road trips, or remote travel destinations.

After Your Trip:

1. Reflect and Share: Reflect on your travel experiences and take note of what worked well and what could be improved for future trips. Share your insights and

recommendations with fellow travelers, online communities, and advocacy groups to help others with similar dietary restrictions.

2. Celebrate Your Success: Celebrate your ability to navigate travel with dietary restrictions and embrace the adventure of exploring new destinations while prioritizing your health and well-being. Remember that with careful planning and flexibility, travel can be both enjoyable and fulfilling, even with dietary limitations.

By incorporating these insights and tips into your travel planning and experiences, you can confidently explore the world while managing your dietary restrictions with ease and enjoyment. Remember to stay flexible, maintain a positive attitude, and embrace the culinary diversity that each destination has to offer.

Chapter Seven: Long-Term Management and Monitoring:

Importance of regular check-ups and follow-ups with healthcare providers

Long-term management and monitoring of gastrointestinal conditions, such as GERD, IBS, gastritis, celiac disease, Crohn's disease, diverticulitis, and pancreatitis, requires ongoing collaboration between patients and healthcare providers. Regular check-ups and follow-ups with healthcare providers play a crucial role in maintaining optimal health, managing symptoms, and preventing complications. Here's why they are important:

1. Assessment of Disease Progression: Regular check-ups allow healthcare providers to assess the progression of the gastrointestinal condition and monitor any changes in symptoms, severity, or complications. This helps identify potential flare-ups or disease exacerbations early on, allowing for timely intervention and management.

2. Medication Management: Healthcare providers can review current medication regimens, adjust dosages as needed, and prescribe new medications to better manage symptoms and improve quality of life. They can also monitor for potential side effects or interactions with other medications.

3. Nutritional Evaluation: Patients with gastrointestinal conditions may have specific dietary needs or restrictions that require ongoing monitoring and support. Healthcare providers, including registered dietitians, can assess nutritional status, address deficiencies, and provide guidance on dietary modifications to optimize gastrointestinal health.

4. Lifestyle Counseling: Healthcare providers can offer personalized lifestyle counseling and recommendations to help patients adopt healthy habits, such as stress management techniques, regular exercise, smoking cessation, and alcohol moderation. These lifestyle modifications can contribute to symptom relief and disease management.

5. Screening for Complications: Certain gastrointestinal conditions, such as Crohn's disease and celiac disease, are associated with an increased risk of complications such as malnutrition, intestinal strictures, and

colorectal cancer. Regular check-ups may include screening tests, imaging studies, or endoscopic procedures to detect and monitor for potential complications.

6. Psychosocial Support: Living with a chronic gastrointestinal condition can take a toll on patients' mental and emotional well-being. Healthcare providers can offer psychosocial support, counseling, and referrals to mental health professionals as needed to address anxiety, depression, stress, and coping difficulties.

7. Patient Education and Empowerment: Regular follow-ups provide opportunities for patient education, empowerment, and engagement in self-management strategies. Healthcare providers can educate patients about their condition, treatment options, symptom management techniques, and resources for support.

8. Treatment Optimization: Over time, treatment approaches for gastrointestinal conditions may need to be adjusted or optimized based on individual response, disease progression, and evolving clinical guidelines. Regular check-ups allow healthcare providers to reassess treatment

goals, modify treatment plans, and explore new therapeutic options as needed.

9. Preventive Care: In addition to managing existing gastrointestinal conditions, regular check-ups also encompass preventive care measures, such as vaccinations, screenings for other gastrointestinal disorders or comorbidities, and health promotion activities to maintain overall wellness.

By prioritizing regular check-ups and follow-ups with healthcare providers, patients with gastrointestinal conditions can receive comprehensive, multidisciplinary care that addresses their medical, nutritional, psychological, and lifestyle needs. These proactive measures contribute to better disease management, improved quality of life, and enhanced long-term outcomes for patients living with chronic gastrointestinal conditions.

Adjusting treatment plans as needed over time

Adjusting treatment plans over time is a common and necessary aspect of managing gastrointestinal conditions effectively. Here's why it's important and how it's typically done:

Importance of Adjusting Treatment Plans:

1. Disease Progression: Gastrointestinal conditions can vary in severity and may progress or change over time. Adjusting treatment plans allows healthcare providers to address evolving symptoms, complications, or disease activity.

2. Response to Treatment: Patients may respond differently to various treatments, medications, and lifestyle modifications. Adjustments may be needed to optimize treatment efficacy, minimize side effects, and improve symptom control.

3. Changing Needs: Patients' needs, preferences, and circumstances may change over time, requiring modifications to treatment plans to accommodate new priorities, challenges, or goals.

4. New Research and Guidelines: Advances in medical research and clinical guidelines may lead to changes in recommended treatments, diagnostic approaches, or management strategies for gastrointestinal conditions. Regular updates ensure that patients receive the most current and evidence-based care.

How Treatment Plans are Adjusted:

1. Regular Follow-Up Visits: Schedule regular follow-up visits with your healthcare provider to monitor your condition, assess treatment response, and discuss any changes in symptoms, medication tolerance, or quality of life.

2. Symptom Assessment: Provide detailed feedback about your symptoms, including their type, frequency, severity, and duration. This information helps healthcare providers evaluate the effectiveness of current treatments and identify areas for adjustment.

3. Medication Review: Review your current medication regimen with your healthcare provider to assess its efficacy, safety, and tolerability. Discuss any concerns or side effects you may be experiencing and explore alternative medications or dosage adjustments as needed.

4. Diagnostic Testing: Consider additional diagnostic testing, such as blood tests, imaging studies, endoscopic procedures, or functional testing, to evaluate disease activity, monitor complications, or assess treatment response over time.

5. Lifestyle Modifications: Evaluate your current lifestyle habits, including diet, exercise, stress management, sleep hygiene, and smoking or alcohol use. Make adjustments as needed to optimize symptom management and support overall health.

6. Collaborative Decision-Making: Engage in collaborative decision-making with your healthcare provider to develop a tailored treatment plan that aligns with your individual needs, preferences, and treatment goals. Explore different treatment options, discuss potential risks and benefits, and weigh the pros and cons together.

7. Long-Term Monitoring: Establish a long-term monitoring plan to track your progress, evaluate treatment outcomes, and identify any changes or trends over time. Regular reassessment ensures that your treatment plan remains effective and responsive to your evolving needs.

Patient Engagement and Advocacy:

1. Active Participation: Take an active role in your healthcare by advocating for your needs, asking questions, expressing concerns, and providing feedback about your treatment experiences.

2. Open Communication: Maintain open and honest communication with your healthcare provider, sharing any changes in symptoms, treatment preferences, or quality of life concerns that may arise.

3. Patient Education: Stay informed about your condition, treatment options, and self-management strategies through patient education resources, support groups, and reputable medical websites. Empower yourself with knowledge to make informed decisions about your care.

By actively participating in the treatment adjustment process, collaborating with your healthcare provider, and staying engaged in your own care, you can optimize the management of your gastrointestinal condition and achieve better long-term outcomes. Remember that treatment plans may need to be adapted over time based on your individual response, disease course, and evolving healthcare landscape.

Conclusion

Recap of key points covered in the book

Here's a recap of the key points covered in the book on gastrointestinal health:

1. Understanding Gastrointestinal Disorders: The book provides an overview of common gastrointestinal disorders, including GERD, IBS, gastritis, celiac disease, Crohn's disease, diverticulitis, and pancreatitis. Each condition is explained in terms of its symptoms, triggers, and impact on daily life.

2. Importance of Managing Symptoms: Emphasizing the importance of symptom management, the book offers practical tips and strategies for coping with symptoms and improving quality of life. It highlights the role of lifestyle modifications, stress management, and dietary considerations in symptom control.

3. Dietary Modifications: Detailed dietary modifications are discussed for each gastrointestinal disorder, including foods to avoid and foods to include. The book offers recipes, meal plans, and cooking tips tailored

to accommodate specific dietary needs and preferences.

4. Medications and Supplements: An overview of common medications prescribed for gastrointestinal disorders is provided, along with potential side effects and interactions to be aware of. The role of supplements, such as probiotics and digestive enzymes, in managing symptoms is also explored.

5. Coping Strategies and Emotional Support: The book addresses the emotional impact of living with a chronic digestive condition and offers coping strategies, stress management techniques, and sources of emotional support for patients and caregivers.

6. Practical Tips for Everyday Living: Practical tips for managing symptoms at home and on the go are discussed, including meal planning, stress reduction, sleep hygiene, and staying hydrated. Strategies for navigating social situations and dining out with dietary restrictions are also provided.

7. Long-Term Management and Monitoring: The importance of regular check-ups and follow-ups with healthcare providers for long-term management is highlighted. The book emphasizes the need for ongoing symptom

monitoring, treatment adjustments, and patient engagement in healthcare decision-making.

Overall, the book serves as a comprehensive guide for individuals living with gastrointestinal disorders, offering practical advice, expert insights, and supportive resources to help them effectively manage their condition and improve their overall well-being.

Encouragement

As you close this chapter and continue on your journey towards better gastrointestinal health, I want to leave you with a few words of encouragement and empowerment.

First and foremost, remember that you are stronger and more resilient than you may realize. While living with gastrointestinal conditions can present its challenges, it's important to recognize the incredible strength and courage you possess in facing these challenges head-on.

You have the power to take control of your health and make positive changes that will benefit you in the long run. Whether it's adopting healthier lifestyle habits, seeking support from healthcare professionals, or connecting with others who understand what you're going through, know that there are countless resources and options available to you.

Embrace each day as an opportunity to learn, grow, and thrive despite any obstacles you may encounter. Celebrate your victories, no matter how small, and be kind to yourself on days when things don't go as planned.

Above all, remember that you are not alone on this journey. Reach out for support when you need it, lean on your loved ones for encouragement, and never underestimate the power of community and connection in overcoming life's challenges.

You are capable, you are resilient, and you are deserving of a life filled with health, happiness, and fulfillment. Keep moving forward with courage, confidence, and a steadfast belief in your ability to overcome any obstacle that comes your way. You've got this!

Additional Resources: - List of reputable websites, books, and organizations for further information and support

Here are some additional resources, including reputable websites, books, and organizations, where you can find further information and support for managing gastrointestinal conditions:

Websites:

1. Crohn's & Colitis Foundation: Provides comprehensive information, resources, and support for individuals living with Crohn's disease and ulcerative colitis. Website: [crohnscolitisfoundation.org](https://www.crohnscolitisfoundation.org/)

2. International Foundation for Gastrointestinal Disorders (IFFGD): Offers educational resources, online support groups, and advocacy initiatives for individuals with functional gastrointestinal and motility disorders. Website: iffgd.org

3. Celiac Disease Foundation: Dedicated to raising awareness, providing support, and

advancing research for individuals with celiac disease and gluten-related disorders.
Website: celiac.org

4. National Institute of Diabetes and Digestive and Kidney Diseases (NIDDK): Provides evidence-based information, research updates, and resources on various digestive diseases and conditions. Website: [niddk.nih.gov](https://www.niddk.nih.gov/)

5. American Gastroenterological Association (AGA): Offers educational materials, clinical guidelines, and patient resources related to gastrointestinal health and digestive disorders.
Website: [gastro.org](https://www.gastro.org/)

Books:

1. "The Complete Low-FODMAP Diet: A Revolutionary Plan for Managing IBS and Other Digestive Disorders" by Sue Shepherd and Peter Gibson
2. "The Acid Watcher Diet: A 28-Day Reflux Prevention and Healing Program" by Dr. Jonathan Aviv
3. "Breaking the Vicious Cycle: Intestinal Health Through Diet" by Elaine Gottschall
4. "The First Year: Crohn's Disease and Ulcerative Colitis: An Essential Guide for the

Newly Diagnosed" by Jill Sklar and Ann Steinhart

Organizations:

1. Beyond Celiac: Advocates for celiac disease awareness, research, and support. Website: [beyondceliac.org](https://www.beyondceliac.org/)
2. Digestive Health Alliance (DHA): Aims to improve the quality of life for individuals affected by digestive disorders through education, support, and advocacy. Website: iffgd.org/dha
3. The Gastroparesis Patient Association for Cures and Treatments (G-PACT): Provides support, education, and advocacy for individuals living with gastroparesis. Website: [g-pact.org](https://www.g-pact.org/)

These resources offer valuable information, support, and community for individuals and caregivers affected by gastrointestinal conditions. Remember to verify the credibility of any information you find and consult with healthcare professionals for personalized advice and treatment recommendations.